I0695545

Table of Contents

Bone marrow is soft, gelatinous tissue that fills the medullary cavities, or the centers of bones. The two types of bone marrow are red bone marrow, known as myeloid tissue, and yellow bone marrow, known as fatty tissue.

Both types of bone marrow are enriched with blood vessels and capillaries.

Bone marrow makes more than 220 billion new blood cells every day. Most blood cells in the body develop from cells in the bone marrow.

Bone marrow stem cells

Bone marrow contains two types of stem cells: mesenchymal and hematopoietic.

Red bone marrow consists of a delicate, highly vascular fibrous tissue containing hematopoietic stem cells. These are blood-forming stem cells.

Yellow bone marrow contains mesenchymal stem cells, or marrow stromal cells. These produce fat, cartilage, and bone.

Stem cells are immature cells that can turn into a number of different types of cells.

Hematopoietic stem cells in the bone marrow give rise to two main types of cells: myeloid and lymphoid lineages. These include monocytes, macrophages, neutrophils, basophils, eosinophils, erythrocytes, dendritic cells, and megakaryocytic, or platelets, as well as T cells, B cells, and natural killer (NK) cells.

The different types of hematopoietic stem cells vary in their regenerative capacity and potency. They can be multipotent, oligopotent, or unipotent, depending on how many types of cells they can create.

Pluripotent hematopoietic stem cells have renewal and differentiation properties. They can reproduce another cell identical to themselves, and they can generate one or more subsets of more mature cells.

The process of developing different blood cells from these pluripotent stem cells is known as hematopoiesis. It is these stem cells that are needed in bone marrow transplants.

Stem cells constantly divide and produce new cells. Some new cells remain as stem cells, while others go through a series of maturing stages, as precursor or blast cells, before becoming formed, or mature, blood cells. Stem cells rapidly multiply to make millions of blood cells each day.

Blood cells have a limited life span. This is around 120 days for red blood cells. The body is constantly replacing them. The production of healthy stem cells is vital.

The blood vessels act as a barrier to prevent immature blood cells from leaving bone marrow.

Only mature blood cells contain the membrane proteins required to attach to and pass through the blood vessel endothelium. Hematopoietic stem cells can cross the bone marrow barrier, however. Healthcare professionals may harvest these from peripheral, or circulating, blood.

BREAKFAST

1. Ultimate Breakfast Burrito

Prep Time: 20 minutes

Cook Time: 20 minutes

Total Time: 40 minutes

Servings: 9

Ingredients

- 1 tablespoon olive oil
- 2 cups bell pepper (finely chopped)
- 1 tablespoon olive oil
- 8 eggs
- salt & pepper
- 1 cup ham (cut into small cubes)
- 2 cups shredded cheese
- 8 tortillas (large; 12 inch)
- ½ cup salsa

Instructions

1. Heat 1 tablespoon of olive oil over medium heat in a non-stick pan. Add the bell pepper and cook for 5-7 minutes, until soft. Transfer to a plate and allow to cool slightly.

2. In a large bowl or measuring cup, beat the eggs. Stir in the salt and pepper. Add the remaining 1 tablespoon of olive oil to the pan and then add the eggs. Cook, scrambling with a spatula, for 3-4 minutes until cooked through. Set aside to cool slightly.

3. To assemble breakfast burritos: place a large tortilla on a cutting board. Top with ⅛ of the egg mixture, a few spoons of bell peppers, ham and shredded cheese, and a spoonful of salsa.

4. Roll burritos by folding over the sides, then the top. Roll tightly, then wrap in plastic wrap.

5. Storage

6. Store in the fridge for up to 3 days. Freeze by placing wrapped burritos in a larger reusable bag or storage container for up to 3 months.

7. To Re-Heat

8. Thaw in the fridge overnight or on low power in the microwave.

9. Crisp up on an indoor grill or in a frying pan.

2. Apple & Cinnamon Baked Oatmeal

Prep Time 10 minutes

Cook Time 35 minutes

Total Time 45 minutes

Servings:9

Ingredients

- 2 tablespoons Linwoods Flaxseeds with Cinnamon and Apple
- 1 tablespoon ground flaxseeds
- 9 tablespoons water
- 1/3 cup raisins
- 2 cups rolled oats gluten-free (optional)
- 2 cups apples diced
- 2 tablespoons pecan nuts chopped
- 3/4 teaspoon salt
- 1 teaspoon ground cinnamon
- 1/4 teaspoon nutmeg
- 1 1/2 cups almond milk or milk of your choice
- 1/4 cup coconut oil melted

- 1/2 teaspoon vanilla extract
- 3 tablespoons maple syrup

Instructions

1. Preheat your oven to 350°F/175°C.
2. In a small bowl, mix the Linwoods Hemp Protein+, flaxseed and water, let sit for 5 minutes. It will go gloopy and act as an egg replacement. If you can't source this particular protein powder simply replace it with more ground flaxseeds.
3. Soak the raisins in warm water for 5 minutes or until they become plump.
4. In a big bowl combine all dry ingredients including the apples and raisins.
5. In another small bowl mix the wet ingredients until well combined.
6. Add the wet ingredients to the dry ingredients and stir until it starts forming a sticky dough.
7. Fill the mixture into a greased 8x8-inch baking pan and bake for 35minutes or until golden brown.

3. Egg Muffins

Prep Time: 20 minutes

Cook Time: 20 minutes

Servings: 4

Ingredients

Base Recipe:

- 8 eggs
- ½ teaspoon salt
- ½ teaspoon pepper
- 2 cups mixed vegetables cut into small cubes (ie: zucchini, onion, bell
- peppers torn spinach, mushrooms, broccoli florets)
- 1 cups shredded cheese ½ cup reserved for sprinkling muffin tops
- ½ cup all purpose flour see note 1
- ½ teaspoon baking powder see note 2
- Sun Dried Tomato, Spinach & Mushroom Egg Muffins
- ½ cup sun dried tomatoes drained from oil and chopped into small pieces

- 1 ½ cups chopped spinach
- 1 ½ cups chopped mushrooms

Instructions

1. Heat oven to 350°F.
2. Line a standard sized muffin pan with parchment or silicone liners and set aside.
3. In a large bowl, mix together the vegetables, feta (when used), eggs, salt and pepper, until well combined.
4. Stir in the flour and baking powder until completely incorporated.
5. Spoon the mixture into the muffin pan, filling nearly full. Sprinkle tops with reserved cheese.
6. Bake in the pre-heated oven for 20-25 minutes, until muffins are baked through and no longer jiggle.

4. Quiche Recipe with Bacon, Tomato and Green Onion

Prep Time: 15 minutes

Cook Time: 33 minutes

Servings: 8 people

Ingredients

- 6 slices bacon
- 2 medium russet potatoes
- 12 large eggs
- 2 cups cheddar cheese (shredded)
- ½ cup green onion (chopped)
- ½ cup tomato (diced)
- 1/8 tsp sea salt
- 1/8 tsp black pepper

Instructions

1. Preheat oven to 375°F.
2. Place the pan on the stove over medium heat.

3. Chop the bacon and add it to the pan.

4. While the bacon is frying, cut the potatoes into very thin slices.

5. Once the bacon is crispy, remove it from the pan and set aside.

6. Pour out any excess bacon grease that is present. A thin layer of grease should be left to prevent the potato crust from sticking, but you don't need much.

7. Place potato slices in the skillet to form a crust, like this:

8. In a medium bowl, whisk the eggs together.

9. Stir in the shredded cheese, green onion, tomato, salt, and pepper.

10. Crumble the bacon and add it to the egg mixture, then carefully pour the mixture into the skillet over the potatoes.

11. Place skilled in the preheated oven and bake for 20-25 minutes, or until set in the center.

12. To use two 9 inch pie plates rather than the cast iron skillet prepare exactly the same way, greasing the pie plates with bacon drippings and slicing some of the potato slices in half to fit the shorter sides of the pie pan.

13. Place the pie plates in the oven and bake for 15-25 minutes, or until set in the center.

5. Baked Pumpkin Oatmeal Recipe with Vanilla Glaze

Prep Time: 15 minutes

Cook Time: 30 minutes

Servings: 9

Ingredients

For the baked pumpkin oatmeal:

- 2 ½ cups gluten-free rolled oats (I use these sprouted rolled oats)
- 1 tsp baking powder (how to make your own baking powder)
- 2 tbsp homemade pumpkin pie spice
- ¼ cup dates (chopped)
- 1 cup milk (or almond milk if dairy-free)
- 1 cup pumpkin puree (either homemade or store-bought)
- 4 large eggs
- 2 tbsp butter (melted - can substitute coconut oil if dairy-free)

- ½ cup maple syrup

- 2 tsp vanilla extract (how to make your own vanilla extract)

For the vanilla glaze:

- 6 tbsp coconut butter

- 1 tbsp raw honey (or maple syrup)

- ¼ cup water

- ¼ tsp vanilla extract

Instructions

1. To make the pumpkin oatmeal:
2. Preheat the oven to 375°F.
3. Prepare an 8x8 baking dish by greasing with butter, coconut oil, or palm shortening.
4. Place dry ingredients (oats, baking powder, pumpkin spice and dates/raisins) in a large bowl. Stir to combine.
5. In another bowl, whisk together the milk, pumpkin puree, eggs, coconut oil/butter, 1/2 cup maple syrup and 2 teaspoons vanilla.
6. Pour the wet ingredients in with oat mixture and stir until well-combined.

7. Pour the batter into the prepared 8x8 baking dish.

8. Bake in the preheated oven at 375 F for about 30-35 minutes, or until center is set. Let cool for 5 to 10 minutes.

9. To make the glaze topping:

10. Add the coconut butter, honey, water, and vanilla to a small pan.

11. Place over low heat and stir constantly until the texture is smooth and spreadable, adding more water if necessary.

12. When the pumpkin oatmeal has cooled a little, drizzle the glaze over the top, then slice and serve.

6. Cinnamon Apple Fritters

Prep Time: 10 minutes

Cook Time: 15 minutes

Servings: 4

Ingredients

For Apples:

- 3 large apples (peeled, cored, and sliced)
- 1 tsp cinnamon
- 1 tbsp maple sugar (or coconut sugar)
- ¼ tsp lemon juice
- For Batter:
- 1 egg
- ⅓ cup arrowroot flour
- ½ tsp maple sugar (or coconut sugar)
- 1 tbsp maple syrup
- ¼ tsp cinnamon
- ¼ tsp nutmeg
- 1 pinch sea salt
- avocado oil (or sub coconut oil/ghee for frying)

- For Glaze (optional):
- 1 cup powdered sugar
- 1 to 2 tbsp almond milk
- ¼ tsp cinnamon

Instructions

For the Apples:

1. Peel, core, and slice the apples into 5 slices each.
2. In a medium size bowl, combine the apple slices with lemon juice, cinnamon, maple or coconut sugar.
3. Gently mix until all the apple slices are evenly coated.
4. Set the apples aside.
5. For the Batter:
6. Place 1 inch of coconut oil for frying in a skillet and heat.
7. While the oil is heating, in another bowl prepare the batter by combining and mixing together the arrowroot, maple sugar, cinnamon, salt, and nutmeg.
8. Add the eggs and maple syrup and stir to combine.
9. When the oil is hot, work in batches dipping each apple slice into the batter and dropping gently into the oil to fry.

10. Cook 1-2 minutes on each side then transfer to a paper towel lined plate.

11. Repeat until all the apples are cooked.

12. For the Glaze:

13. Whisk all ingredients together in a small bowl until combined.

14. Let apples cool slightly, then enjoy with the optional glaze listed above for breakfast or a scoop of vanilla ice cream for dessert!

7. Easy Gluten-Free Waffle Recipe Made with Almond Flour

Prep Time: 10 minutes

Total Time: 10 minutes

Servings: 4 waffles

Equipment:

- large bowl
- Waffle Maker
- medium bowl
- Whisk or wooden spoon

Ingredients

- 2 cups blanched almond flour (packed)
- 1 ½ cups arrowroot flour (tapioca starch will also work)
- 4 tsp baking powder ½ tsp sea salt
- 4 large eggs
- ⅔ cup melted butter (substitute melted coconut oil or avocado oil if dairy-free)
- ⅔ cup milk (buttermilk, almond milk, coconut milk and water will also work)

- ½ tsp vanilla extract

Instructions

1. Preheat your waffle iron.
2. Combine dry ingredients (almond flour, arrowroot flour, baking powder and salt) in a large bowl.
3. In a separate bowl, whisk together the wet ingredients – eggs, butter/oil, milk, vanilla.
4. Add the wet ingredients to the dry ingredients and whisk together until well-combined.
5. Cook waffles in the preheated waffle iron according to the manufacturer's instructions.
6. If needed, reheat the waffles in a toaster.

8. Zucchini Fritters

Prep Time15 minutes

Cook Time10 minutes

Servings: 9

Equipment

- grater
- Cheesecloth or a thin, clean kitchen towel (Paper towels will also work, but you have to be careful not to break them when squeezing the excess liquid out of the zucchini)

Ingredients

- 5 cups grated zucchini
- 1 tsp sea salt
- 3 tbsp cassava flour (or Bob's Red Mill Gluten-Free All-Purpose Flour)
- ⅓ cup grated parmesan cheese (plus more for garnish if desired)
- 1 large egg, beaten
- 1 tbsp dried parsley

- 1 tsp garlic powder

- 1 tsp onion powder

- ¼ tsp black pepper

- ½ tsp baking powder

- coconut oil or ghee for frying

- sour cream or Greek yogurt for topping (optional)

Instructions

1. Add the shredded zucchini to a large colander and sprinkle the salt over it. Toss to combine and then place the colander in the kitchen sink for ten minutes.

2. Remove the zucchini from the colander and place it in the center of a piece of cheesecloth, a clean lightweight kitchen towel, or a few layers of paper towels. Squeeze the zucchini over the kitchen sink to drain as much excess moisture as possible. Set aside the zucchini.

3. Add the cassava flour, parmesan, egg, dried parsley, garlic powder, onion powder, pepper, and baking powder to the bowl and stir until everything is well-combined. Add in the shredded zucchini and stir again until it is fully mixed in.

4. In a large skillet, heat 2 tablespoons coconut oil or ghee over medium-high heat.

5. When the skillet is hot, reduce to medium heat, then scoop out two tablespoons of the fritter mixture and form it into a ball. Place it in the pan and press it flat using a spatula. Continue adding patties to the pan – spacing each one about one inch apart – until the pan is full.

6. Fry for 2-3 minutes – or until the patties golden-brown on one side – then flip them and cook on the other side.

7. Continue the process until all the fritter mixture is used. Add coconut oil/ghee as needed.

8. Serve hot with a dollop of sour cream or Greek yogurt if desired.

9. Fried Rice with Cauliflower

Prep Time10 minutes

 Cook Time15 minutes

Servings: 3

Ingredients

- 3 cups cauliflower (or 2-3 cups cooked)
- 2-3 tbsp olive oil (or butter)
- 3 garlic cloves (minced)
- 1 small onion (diced)
- 1 cup green peas
- 2 carrots (diced)
- 2 cup broccoli florets (in small pieces)
- 6 eggs
- 1-2 tbsp naturally fermented soy sauce (or coconut aminos)
- sea salt (to taste)
- black pepper (to taste)

Instructions

1. Cut cauliflower into chunks and then pulse a few times in your food processor. You want the pieces to resemble little peas (or little grains of rice).

2. In a large pan on medium heat, add butter or olive oil, minced garlic, and diced onions; cook for about 3-4 minutes. Add in carrot, broccoli, and peas; cook for 5-7 minutes (placing a lid on the pan will help cook the veggies quicker if you have a little one that likes softer veggies versus al dente). You may want to add more butter or olive oil at this point.

3. Meanwhile in a bowl, scramble 6 eggs and season them with salt and pepper. Once the veggies are done cooking, make a little hole in the middle of them and pour your eggs. Scramble the eggs like you normally would. Next, add in the cauliflower and soy sauce; stir until well combined. Let cook for 2-3 minutes, stirring occasionally and remove from the stove.

4. Add more soy sauce/coconut aminos if desired, and season with salt and pepper.

10. Asian Beef Noodle Soup

Prep Time: 10 minutes

Cook Time: 25 minutes

Servings4 -6 servings

Ingredients

- 2 qts beef broth
- 1 – 1½ lbs flank steak (cut into strips – I've also used strip steak, sirloin and even leftover pieces from a roast)
- 3 – 4 tsps sesame oil
- 4 – 8 cloves garlic (finely chopped)
- 3 – 4 inch piece of fresh ginger (peeled and chopped)
- 1 bok choy (chopped – separate and set aside the green leafy ends from the whiter stalks)
- 1 red pepper (de-seeded and thinly sliced)
- 15 – 20 shiitake mushrooms (sliced – or other mushrooms of your choice)
- 1 pkg soba noodles
- 3 – 4 tbsp soy sauce

Instructions

1. Saute garlic and ginger in half of sesame oil for about 5 minutes.

2. Add beef broth, soy sauce, mushrooms, red pepper and bok choy stalks to broth and simmer for 5-10 more minutes. Add the bok choy greens in the last minute as they'll cook much quicker than the stalks.

3. While all this is simmering, prepare noodles according to package directions, drain in cold water.

4. Salt and pepper both sides of the flank steak. Lightly sear the steak in the rest of the sesame oil, 2-3 minutes per side so that the outside is browned but the inside is still pink. It's best to undercook it because it will cook a bit more when you add the hot broth. Remove from heat and slice the steak, across the grain, into strips of any size you prefer.

5. Put several beef strips and a handful of noodles in serving bowls and ladle broth with vegetables over.

6. Add more soy sauce if needed, to taste.

11. Apple Sandwiches

Servings: 6 sandwiches

Ingredients

- 2 medium apples (and an apple corer)
- 1 ½ cups chicken (shredded – about ¼ pound)
- 1 lemon
- 6 slices cheese (I use raw cheddar)
- sliced onion
- mayo (I use my homemade recipe)
- 6 slices bacon (optional – I often have some leftover from breakfast that I throw on top of the cheese)
- 6 leaves lettuce (optional)

Instructions

1. Core apples using an apple corer and slice them into approximately 12 pieces – I sometimes end up with a few extra pieces, which I just serve on the side.

2. Cut the lemon into four pieces. Pick up one piece and give it a gently squeeze to release some of the juice. Rub the lemon on the outside of the apple to prevent browning and repeat

3. Put half of the apple slices on a plate and set aside the other half for later.

4. Divide the chicken equally between the slices on the plate.

5. Divide the cheese equally between the slices on the plate, then add additional toppings if desired.

6. Top the apple slices, bacon/deli meat, cheese and any additional toppins with the remaining apple slices to complete your sandwich, then serve.

12. Turkey Taco Meal Bowls

Prep Time: 20 mins

Cook Time: 50 mins

Servings: 5

Ingredients

Rice

- ¾ cup brown rice (uncooked; may be swapped for quinoa or long grain white rice)
- ⅛ tsp salt
- 1 lime (zested)
- Turkey
- ¾ lb lean ground turkey (beef or chicken may be swapped)
- 2 tablespoons homemade taco seasoning
- ⅔ cup water

Salsa

- 1 pint cherry tomatoes (halved)
- 1 jalapeno (finely chopped)
- ¼ cup red onion (finely chopped)

- ½ lime (juiced)
- ⅛ teaspoon salt

Other:

- 12 oz can corn kernels (341 mL; drained)
- ½ cup mozzarella (shredded)

Instructions

1. Cook brown rice according to package directions, adding the lime zest and salt to the cooking water. Allow to cool
2. slightly before portioning out.
3. Add turkey to a medium pan and cook over medium heat, breaking it up with a spatula until no longer pink (approximately 10 minutes).
4. Sprinkle the taco seasoning over the cooked meat, then add the water. Stir and simmer for a couple of minutes, until sauce has thickened.
5. Remove from heat and allow to cool slightly before portioning out.
6. Combine all salsa ingredients and toss together.
7. To assemble lunch bowls, divide ingredients evenly between four 2-cup capacity meal prep containers.

8. Storage

9. Store in the fridge for up to 4 days.

10. You may serve cold or warm up in the microwave before enjoying

13. Honey Sesame Chicken Lunch Bowls

Prep Time: 10 minutes

Cook Time: 20 minutes

Servings: 6

Ingredients

Honey Sesame Sauce:

- ¼ cup chicken stock or water
- ¼ cup reduced sodium soy sauce
- ¼ cup honey (or maple syrup)
- 1 tablespoon sesame oil
- ½ teaspoon red pepper flakes
- 1 teaspoon cornstarch

Chicken Lunch Bowls:

- ¾ cup rice (uncooked; or roughly 2 cups cooked)
- 2 tablespoons olive oil (divided)
- 3 cups broccoli (chopped into small pieces)
- 3 cups snap peas (ends trimmed)
- 2 large chicken breasts (cut into 1 inch cubes)
- salt & pepper

- sesame seeds (garnish)

Instructions

1. Shake together all honey sesame sauce ingredients and set aside.
2. Cook rice according to package instructions. Divide between 4 storage containers.
3. Heat 1 tablespoon olive oil in a large pan. Add broccoli and snap peas. Cook for 5-7 minutes, until bright green and tender. Add to the rice in the storage containers.
4. Add remaining 1 tablespoon olive oil to pan. Add the chicken to the pan. Season with salt and pepper, and red pepper flakes (if desired). Cook for 7-10 minutes, until cooked through.
5. Add the sauce to the pan and simmer for 2 minutes, until thickened.
6. Add the chicken to the lunch containers and drizzle with sauce. Garnish with sesame seeds if desired.
7. Store in the fridge for up to 4 days. Reheat to serve.

14. Chili Lime Sweet Potato and Chicken Skillet

Prep Time: 15 Minutes

Cook Time: 30 Minutes

Servings: 4

Ingredients

- 1 lb boneless skinless chicken breasts (roughly 2 large chicken breasts; cut into 1-inch cubes)
- 2 tablespoons olive oil
- salt and pepper
- 4 cups sweet potato cubes (cut into 1-cm (½ inch) cubes; approximately 1 large or 2 smaller sweet potatoes)
- 2 bell peppers (cut into ½ inch pieces)
- 1 red onion (1 small onion or ½ large onion; diced)
- 2 tablespoons chili powder
- 2 teaspoons ground cumin
- ¼ teaspoon salt
- 1 cup chicken stock

- 1 tablespoon lime zest
- 1 can black beans drained (540mL/18 oz)

To Serve

- shredded cheddar cheese
- cilantro leaves
- lime wedges
- greek yogurt or sour cream
- avocado
- tortilla chips

Instructions

1. In a large skillet or pan, heat 1 tablespoon of olive oil over medium heat. Add the chicken, and cook until no longer pink in the middle (roughly 8-10 minutes).
2. Remove the chicken from the pan and place on a clean plate.
3. Add the sweet potato, bell peppers, red onion, chili powder, cumin, salt, chicken stock and lime zest.
4. Cover and bring to a simmer. Simmer (covered) for 15-20 minutes, stirring 2-3 times, until sweet potatoes are soft and cooked through. If the pan becomes dry, add more chicken stock.

5. Add the black beans and cooked chicken breast, and cook 2 or so minutes until heated through.

6. Serve with suggested toppings.

15. Buddha Bowl

Prep Time: 15 Minutes

Cook Time: 25 Minutes

Servings: 3

Ingredients

- Chickpea Buddha Bowls
- ¾ cup uncooked quinoa
- 2 large carrots (peeled & chopped)
- 1 red onion (chopped into 1 inch pieces)
- 2 cups brussels sprouts (outer leaves removed and cut in half)
- 2 tablespoons olive oil
- salt & pepper
- 19 oz can of chickpeas (drained; 15 or 19 oz can)
- Tahini Dressing
- 2 tablespoons tahini
- 2 tablespoons water
- 2 teaspoons maple syrup
- 2 teaspoons lemon juice
- salt

Instructions

1. Cook quinoa according to package directions. Portion out into four 2-cup capacity storage containers and allow to cool.
2. Heat oven to 425°F. Line a baking sheet with parchment and set aside.
3. Toss carrots, onion, brussels sprouts in olive oil and season with salt & pepper.
4. Spread out on the baking sheet and bake in the oven for 15-20 minutes, stirring halfway through, or until veggies are soft.
5. While veggies are baking, shake together all tahini dressing ingredients.
6. Between the four meal prep containers, portion out the chickpeas, veggies, and tahini sauce (you can drizzle right away or add it to a condiment container to add fresh).
7. Storage
8. Store in the fridge for up to 4 days. Reheat until steaming hot, or enjoy cold.

16. Caprese Chicken Salad

Prep Time: 15 Minutes

Cook Time: 25 Minutes

Servings: 5

Ingredients

- ¾ cup quinoa uncooked
- 1 tablespoon olive oil
- 1 tablespoon balsamic vinegar
- 1 lb boneless skinless chicken breasts roughly 2 large chicken breasts; see note 1
- salt & pepper
- 3 cups cherry tomatoes halved
- 1 bunch basil leaves whole but removed from stem; see note 2
- 1 cup baby bocconcini see note 3
- Balsamic Vinaigrette
- 3 tablespoons olive oil
- 3 tablespoons balsamic vinegar
- 1 tablespoon maple syrup
- ¼ teaspoon dijon

- salt & pepper

Instructions

1. Cook quinoa- cook quinoa according to package directions. Allow to cool.

2. Cook chicken- Heat oven to 425°F. Toss 1 lb boneless skinless chicken breast with 1 tablespoon olive oil and 1 tablespoon balsamic vinegar. Transfer to a baking dish, season with salt and pepper and bake for 25 minutes, or until chicken reaches 165°F in the thickest part.

3. Once chicken has rested for at least 10 minutes, slice it against the grain.

4. Shake up vinaigrette- In a salad dressing shaker or mason jar, combine the olive oil, balsamic vinegar, maple syrup, dijon and salt and pepper. Portion out into condiment containers.

5. Portion & store- In four meal prep containers (2 cups or larger), divide up the cooled quinoa, chicken, cherry tomatoes, mozzarella balls, and basil leaves. Store in the fridge for up to 4 days.

6. Serve- When you are ready to serve, tear up the fresh basil leaves, shake up the salad dressing, and drizzle over everything. Toss up the salad, and enjoy!

17. Vegan Moroccan Chickpea Skillet

Prep Time: 15 Minutes

Cook Time: 30 Minutes

Servings: 6

Ingredients

- 15 oz chickpeas (drained & rinsed)
- 19 oz can of diced tomatoes (with juices)
- 1 bell pepper chopped
- 2 cups sweet potato (cut in ½ inch cubes)
- 1 onion chopped
- 1 ½ tablespoons Homemade Moroccan Spice Blend
- ¼ teaspoon salt

To Serve

- ½ lemon (juiced)

- parsley

Instructions

1. Add all ingredients to a large skillet and stir up. Cover and simmer for 30 minutes or until sweet potatoes are cooked through, stirring up occasionally.
2. If you see the skillet becoming dry, add in ½ cup water or stock and cover.
3. Storage
4. Store in the fridge for up to 4 days or the freezer for 1-2 months.
5. To Assemble Ahead And Freeze
6. Combine all ingredients in a good quality gallon-sized freezer bag. Squeeze out as much air as possible and freeze flat for up to 3 months.
7. Thaw completely before cooking in skillet as directed above. Start checking for doneness at 15 minutes.

18. Southwestern Chopped Chicken Salad

Prep Time: 15 Minutes

Cook Time: 25 Minutes

Servings: 4

Ingredients

Chicken:

- ½ teaspoon onion powder
- ½ teaspoon garlic powder
- ½ teaspoon chili powder
- ½ teaspoon ground cumin
- ½ teaspoon salt
- ½ teaspoon red pepper flakes
- 1 tablespoon olive oil
- 2 large chicken breasts 12-14 oz

Salad:

- 4 cups romaine lettuce chopped into bite-sized pieces
- 1 cup cherry tomatoes halved
- ½ cup red onions chopped
- ½ red bell pepper chopped

- 1 cup corn kernels drained and rinsed
- 19 oz can of black beans drained & rinsed

To Serve

- Litehouse Homestyle Ranch Dressing roughly ½ cup; 2 tablespoons per lunch bowl
- ½ cup tortilla strips

Instructions

1. Heat oven to 425°.
2. Mix together all spices.
3. Place chicken breasts in a small baking dish and drizzle with olive oil. Sprinkle with spice mixture, turn chicken over and sprinkle the other side until coated.
4. Bake in the pre-heated oven for 10 minutes, flip, and bake for another 10-15 minutes, until cooked through.
5. Allow to rest at least 10 minutes before chopping into cubes.
6. Divide all salad ingredients amongst four meal prep containers (2 cup capacity). Top with chicken.
7. Store in the fridge for up to 4 days.

8. To ServeDump the contents out into a large bowl, toss with roughly 2 tablespoons of Litehouse Homestyle Ranch Dressing, and sprinkle with tortilla strips.

19. Vegan Sushi Meal

Prep Time: 20 Minutes

Cook Time: 20 Minutes

Servings: 4

Ingredients

Rice

- ¾ cup basmati rice uncooked
- 2 tablespoons seasoned rice vinegar
- 1 sheet seaweed crumbled into small pieces
- Sushi Bowls
- 2 cups edamame shelled, thawed from frozen
- 6 radishes sliced
- 2 carrots cut into matchsticks
- ½ long english cucumber cut into rounds or matchsticks
- Sriracha Mayo
- ¼ cup vegan mayonnaise or regular mayo for non-vegan
- 1 teaspoon sriracha or more if you like it spicy

Instructions

1. Prepare rice - cook rice according to package directions, then allow to cool. Toss with rice vinegar and seaweed.

2. Sriracha mayo - in a small bowl, stir together the mayo and sriracha. Portion out into condiment containers and add into meal prep containers.

3. Portion - portion out rice into four 2-cup capacity storage containers. Portion out edamame, radishes, carrots, and cucumber between the meal prep containers

20. Kale Barley Salad with Feta and A Honey-Lemon Vinaigrette

Prep Time: 20 Minutes

Cook Time: 50 Minutes

Servings: 6

Ingredients

Salad

- ½ cup pearl barley uncooked; just over 1 cup cooked
- 4 cups kale loosely packed;, stems removed, and cut into small ribbons
- ⅓ cup feta crumbled
- 15 oz chickpeas drained & rinsed
- 1 avocado cubed
- 2-3 tablespoons sunflower seeds
- 2 tablespoons red onion finely diced

Vinaigrette

- 2 tablespoons olive oil
- 2 tablespoons white wine vinegar

- 1 teaspoon fresh lemon juice
- ½ teaspoon lemon zest
- 2 teaspoons honey

Instructions

1. Cook Barley - Cook pearl barley according to package directions. Set aside to cool.
2. Prepare Kale - Wash and chop kale. Give it a massage for 1-2 minutes to remove some of the bitterness.
3. Combine Dressing - Whisk together the vinaigrette ingredients.
4. Toss Together Salad- Once barley is cool, toss with the kale, vinaigrette and remaining ingredients. Enjoy!

21.Buffalo Chicken Stuffed Sweet Potatoes

Prep Time: 10 minutes

Cook Time: 40 minutes

Servings: 4

Ingredients

- 4 medium sweet potatoes
- 3 cups cooked and shredded chicken breast (or leftover rotisserie chicken that has been shredded)
- 3 tbsp hot sauce (I use this brand because it has a clean ingredient list and it's GOOD)
- ¼ cup butter
- ½ tsp smoked paprika
- 1 tsp garlic powder (divided)
- ⅔ cup sour cream
- ¾ tsp dried parsley
- ¾ tsp dried dill

- ¼ tsp unrefined sea salt

- ½ cup cheese (grated - optional topping)

- ¼ cup green onions (chopped - optional topping)

- 3 tbsp milk (optional - if you prefer a thick and creamy ranch topping skip the milk. If you prefer a pourable ranch-style dressing, you'll use the milk to thin out the sour cream until it reaches your desired consistency)

Instructions

1. Preheat oven to 400°F. If needed, wash and dry the sweet potatoes. Using a fork, poke 4-5 sets of holes in the skin, then place on a baking sheet and pop in the oven for about 40 minutes to an hour.

2. While the potatoes are cooking, mix together the sour cream, parsley, dill, salt and ½ teaspoon of garlic powder. If you prefer a thick and creamy topping, set it in the fridge for later use. If you prefer a thinner, more pourable topping, add a few tablespoons of milk until the desired consistency is reached.

3. Around the 40 minute mark, check on the sweet potatoes. You'll know they're ready when you can slide a fork in and the flesh is very soft.

4. When the sweet potatoes are ready, turn the oven off and let them sit in the oven while you prepare the buffalo chicken. In a saucepan, combine hot sauce, butter, smoked paprika and ½ teaspoon garlic powder over medium heat. When the butter is melted, stir to combine the ingredients and add the chicken in. When the chicken is warm, remove the sweet potatoes from the oven and stuff the chicken in the sweet potatoes, dividing equally. Top with ranch dip/dressing and cheese or green onion if using.

22. Italian Oven Baked Meatballs

Prep Time15 Minutes

Cook Time20 Minutes

Servings: 2

Equipment:

- large mixing bowl
- 2 rimmed baking sheets
- oven

Ingredients

- 2 pounds ground turkey, ground pork, ground beef or a mixture of ground meats
- 1 cup shredded carrot
- 1 cup minced onion
- 1½ cups shredded zucchini
- ½ cup finely chopped kale (de-stemmed)
- 1 tsp Italian seasoning
- ¾ tsp sea salt
- ½ tsp freshly ground black pepper
- ¼ tsp garlic powder

- chopped fresh parsley for topping (optional)
- parmesan cheese for topping (optional)

Instructions

1. Preheat oven to 375°F.
2. In a large mixing bowl, mix the veggies, spices, salt and pepper. Add in the meat and mix everything together with clean hands.
3. Form the meat mixture into 1 – 1.5 inch balls and place meatballs on two rimmed baking sheets that have been lined with parchment paper. Make sure there is a little space between each one so that they can cook evenly.
4. Bake meatballs for 20-25 minutes, or until inside is no longer pink. If you're using ground turkey and want them to be a little golden brown on top, you can turn on the broiler and for a few minutes to brown just before you remove them from the oven.

23. Healthy Shrimp Chowder

Prep Time: 10 Minutes

Cook Time: 30 Minutes

Servings: 12 cups

Equipment

- vegetable peeler
- chopping knife
- large stock pot
- stirring spoon

Ingredients

- 2 cups potatoes (or substitute cauliflower)
- 2 tbsp butter
- ½ cup celery
- ⅓ cup onion
- ¼ cup dry white wine
- 4 cups chicken or vegetable stock
- 2 cup milk of choice
- 1 lb frozen cooked shrimp (thawed and drained)
- 1 tsp Old Bay seasoning

- ½ tsp dijon mustard

- 1 tbsp lemon juice

- ½ tsp garlic powder

- 1 tsp sea salt

- 8 oz cream cheese

- hot sauce (optional)

Instructions

1. Peel and dice potatoes or chop cauliflower into bite size pieces.

2. In a large stock pot, melt butter over medium heat.

3. Add the potatoes or cauliflower and cook, stirring occasionally until they start to soften, about 8-10 minutes.

4. While the potatoes/cauliflower are cooking, slice the celery and finely dice the onion.

5. Add the celery and onion to the stock pot and cook, stirring occasionally, an additional 8-10 minutes.

6. Add the white wine, scraping the bottom of the pot.

7. Reduce the heat to low and add all the remaining ingredients, heating and stirring occasionally until heated through.

8. If desired, sprinkle with hot sauce to serve.

24. Sheet Pan Chicken Fajitas

Prep Time: 10 Minutes

Cook Time: 25 Minutes

Servings: 6

Equipment

- rimmed baking sheet

Ingredients

- Fajita Seasoning + Oil Mixture
- 1 tbsp chili powder
- 1 tbsp ground cumin
- 2 tsp garlic powder
- 1 tsp paprika
- ¾ tsp oregano
- 1 tsp sea salt
- ¼ tsp black pepper
- pinch cayenne pepper (optional)
- ¼ cup avocado oil or olive oil
- Meat + Veggies Mix
- 1 red bell pepper (sliced into 1/4 inch slices)

- 1 yellow bell pepper (sliced into 1/4 inch slices)

- 1 green bell pepper (sliced into 1/4 inch slices)

- 1 small red or yellow onion (sliced into 1/4 inch slices)

- 1½ pounds chicken breasts (cut into thin strips)

- Topping & Side Ideas

- 2 tbsp lime juice (plus extra lime wedges if desired)

- sour cream

- cilantro

- homemade tortillas

- Mexican rice

Instructions

1. Preheat oven to 375F.

2. In a large bowl, add the oil, chili powder, cumin, garlic powder, paprika, salt, oregano, black pepper, and cayenne (if using). Stir until well combined.

3. Add veggie slices and chicken strips to the bowl and mix until they are well coated with the oil/spice mixture.

4. Place the chicken and veggies on a baking sheet in an even later.

5. Bake for 25-30 minutes, or until the chicken is fully cooked. Once the chicken is finished cooking, you can

turn your oven to broil and place the pan close to the broiler for 2-5 minutes. This step is optional, but I like it because it browns the chicken and adds color to the veggies.

6. Remove the pan from the oven. Sprinkle with lime juice if using, then serve.

25. Paprika Chicken Sheet Pan

Prep Time: 5 Minutes

Cook Time: 25 Minutes

Servings: 3

Ingredients

Rub:

- 2 tablespoons brown sugar
- 1 tablespoon paprika
- ½ teaspoon pepper
- ½ teaspoon salt
- ¼ teaspoon cayenne *omit for a non-spicy version

Sheet Pan:

- 2 large chicken breasts whole
- 2 tablespoons olive oil
- 1.5 lb baby potatoes quartered
- 2 bell peppers chopped
- 1 zucchini chopped
- 1 cup cherry tomatoes whole
- To Serve:

- 2 tablespoons fresh oregano chopped
- Coarse sea salt to taste

Instructions

1. Heat oven to 425°F. Line two baking sheets with parchment paper.
2. In a small bowl, stir together the rub. Rub each chicken breast with 1 tablespoon of the rub, then place them on the baking sheet.
3. In a large bowl, toss the baby potatoes with 1 tablespoon of olive oil. Add 2 tablespoons of reserved rub mixture and toss to coat.
4. Arrange the potatoes on one side of each baking sheet.
5. Bake the chicken and potatoes for 10 minutes.
6. While chicken is baking, toss the bell peppers and zucchini with the other tablespoon of olive oil and additional 1 tablespoon of rub (or whatever is left).
7. After 10 minutes, flip the chicken and arrange the bell peppers and zucchini on the empty side of the baking sheet. Return to the oven for 10 minutes
8. Add the cherry tomatoes to the pan and cook for 5 more minutes.

9. Remove from oven, sprinkle with fresh oregano and coarse sea salt and serve immediately.

26. Jamaican Chicken Sheet

Prep Time: 15 Minutes

Cook Time: 25 Minutes

Servings: 4

Ingredients

Jamaican Rub

- 1 tablespoon dried thyme leaves
- 1 tablespoon ground allspice
- 2 tablespoon brown sugar
- 1 teaspoon salt
- 1 teaspoon pepper
- 1 tablespoon garlic powder
- 1 teaspoon cinnamon
- ⅛ teaspoon cayenne for mild spice or ¼ teaspoon (for spice-ay!)

Sheet Pan

- 2 large chicken breasts
- 4 cups baby potatoes cut SMALL in 4-6 depending on size of potato

- 2 bell peppers cut into chunks
- 1 red onion cut into chunks
- 1 zucchini cut into small pieces
- To Serve

Instructions

1. Heat oven to 425°F. Line two baking sheets with parchment and set aside.
2. Stir together all rub ingredients.
3. In a medium sized bowl, toss the chicken with 1 tablespoon of olive oil and 1.5 tablespoons of the rub. Make sure they are evenly coated, then arrange on one of the baking sheets.
4. In a separate medium sized bowl, toss the potatoes with 1 tablespoon of olive oil and 2 tablespoons of rub. Arrange on the baking sheet around the chicken.
5. Bake for 10 minutes. Flip the chicken and return the pan to the oven for 15 minutes.
6. Toss the peppers, onion and zucchini in 1 tablespoon of olive oil and 2 tablespoons of the rub. Arrange on the second sheet pan and bake for 15 minutes.
7. While sheet pans are cooking, prepare the mango.

8. Allow the chicken to rest for 5 minutes before serving with the mango.

27. One Pot Pasta with Kale & Goat Cheese

Prep Time: 10 Minutes

Cook Time: 20 Minutes

Servings: 5

Ingredients

- 2 cups dried pasta smaller shapes work well
- 2 cups chicken stock
- ¼ teaspoon salt
- ¼ teaspoon pepper
- ¼ teaspoon red pepper flakes
- 2 chicken breasts cut into ½ inch cubes
- 1 small onion diced
- ⅓ cup goat cheese
- 2 cups Cookin Greens Organic Chopped Kale
- juice from 1 lemon
- Garnish
- ¼ cup pine nuts

Instructions

1. In a medium pot, combine the pasta, chicken stock, salt, pepper, red pepper flakes, chicken breast and onion.
2. Cover the pot, bring to a boil, reduce heat and simmer for 10 minutes, stirring ever 2 or so minutes.
3. At this point the pasta should be al dente. Stir in the lemon juice and Cookin Greens Organic Chopped Kale.
4. Cook, uncovered for 2-4 more minutes, until kale is thawed.
5. Stir in the goat cheese until melted through.
6. Serve immediately, garnished with pine nuts.

28. Lemon Chicken Spaghetti Squash

Prep Time: 30 Minutes

Cook Time: 1hrs 5 Minutes

Servings: 6

Ingredients

- one 3 lb spaghetti squash
- 2 large chicken breasts 14 oz
- 1 tablespoon olive oil
- salt & pepper
- Lemon Garlic Cream Sauce
- ¼ cup onion chopped finely
- 1 tablespoon butter
- 2 garlic cloves minced
- ½ cup chicken stock
- juice of ½ a lemon
- ½ cup cream
- ⅛ teaspoon salt optional; to taste
- Other
- ½ cup shredded cheese I used mozzarella

Instructions

1. Squash & ChickenHeat oven to 350°F.

2. Cut spaghetti squash in half and scoop out seeds. Place face-down in a 9x13 inch baking dish and add ½ cup of water to the base of the dish.

3. Bake in the pre-heated oven for 45-50 minutes, until soft on the inside and a knife inserts into the flesh of the squash easily.

4. While squash is baking, prep the chicken. Toss in olive oil and season with salt & pepper. Bake in the oven for 30 minutes or until cooked through. Allow to cool before cutting into cubes.

5. Lemon Garlic Cream SauceWhile squash and chicken are baking, prep the sauce.

6. In a small saucepan, melt the butter. Add onion and cook for 4-5 minutes, until soft and translucent.

7. Add the garlic and cook for 1 minute.

8. Add the stock and cook for 3-4 minutes, until reduced by about half.

9. Stir in the lemon juice and heavy cream, and heat until just bubbling. Taste and add salt if needed

10. Remove from heat.

11. Spaghetti Squash BoatsOnce squash is cooked through, remove from oven and allow to cool slightly

before shredding into spaghettti-like strands using two forks. Add the chicken, toss to coat. Pour ½ cup of lemon garlic cream sauce over each half of the squash.

12. Return to the oven for 10-15 more minutes.

13. Sprinkle with cheese and bake for 5 more minutes, until melted.

29. Mediterranean Salmon Sheet

Prep Time: 5 Minutes

Cook Time: 30 Minutes

Servings: 4

Ingredients

- ¼ cup balsamic vinegar
- ¼ cup olive oil
- 6 cloves garlic minced
- ½ teaspoon salt
- 1 lb baby potatoes cut into quarters (cut the larger ones into 6)
- 16 oz salmon cut into 4 portions
- 2.5 cups fennel thinly sliced
- 2.5 cups brussels sprouts halved
- 1 small red onion cut into wedges

To Serve:

- ½ cup feta cheese crumbled
- 2 tablespoons parsley

Instructions

1. Heat oven to 425°F. Line two baking sheets with parchment paper and set aside.
2. Shake together the balsamic vinegar, olive oil, garlic and salt.
3. Toss the potatoes in ⅓ of the mixture and arrange on one of the baking sheets.
4. Bake for 15 minutes, then stir them up and return to the oven.
5. Arrange the salmon on the second baking sheet, drizzle with ⅓ of the balsamic vinegar mixture.
6. Toss the veggies in the remaining balsamic mixture and arrange around the salmon. Bake for 12-15 minutes, until everything is cooked through.
7. Sprinkle with feta cheese and parsley and serve.

30. Sweet Chili Salmon & Broccoli Quinoa Bowl

Prep Time: 10 Minutes

Cook Time: 20 Minutes

Servings: 2

Ingredients

- ¾ cup uncooked quinoa
- Sweet Chili Salmon
- 4 4 oz salmon fillets
- ¼ cup sweet chilli sauce
- 2 tablespoons soy sauce I use reduced sodium
- 2 tablespoons water
- 2 garlic cloves minced
- Roasted Veggies
- 6 oz/170g snow peas roughly 2 cups
- 2 heads of broccoli roughly 4 cups, cut into bite-sized pieces
- 4 teaspoons olive oil
- 2 teaspoons soy sauce

Instructions

1. Cook quinoa according to package directions.
2. While quinoa is cooking, heat oven to 425°F. Line a large baking sheet with parchment and set aside.
3. Salmon:
4. Whisk together the sweet chili sauce, soy sauce, water and garlic. Pour into a 8x8 inch baking dish. Place the salmon, skin side up, on the sauce. Allow to sit while oven heats.
5. When oven is heated, place in the oven and cook for 15-20 minutes, or until cooked through.
6. Roasted Veggies:
7. Place broccoli and snow peas in a large bowl. Toss with the olive oil and soy sauce, until lightly coated.
8. Place in the oven and roast for 10-15 minutes, until cooked through and tender.